Sensei Self Development

Mental Health Chronicles Series

Understanding and Managing Grief

Sensei Paul David

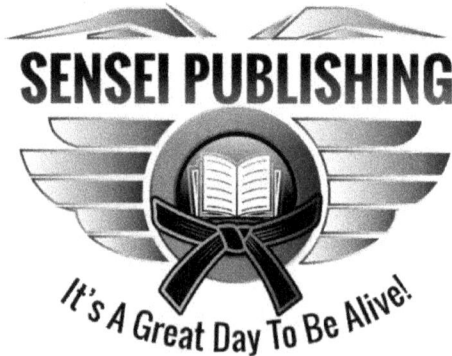

SENSEI PUBLISHING

It's A Great Day To Be Alive!

www.senseipublishing.com

@senseipublishing
#senseipublishing

Get/Share Your FREE SSD Mental Health Chronicles at
www.senseiselfdevelopment.care

or

CLICK HERE

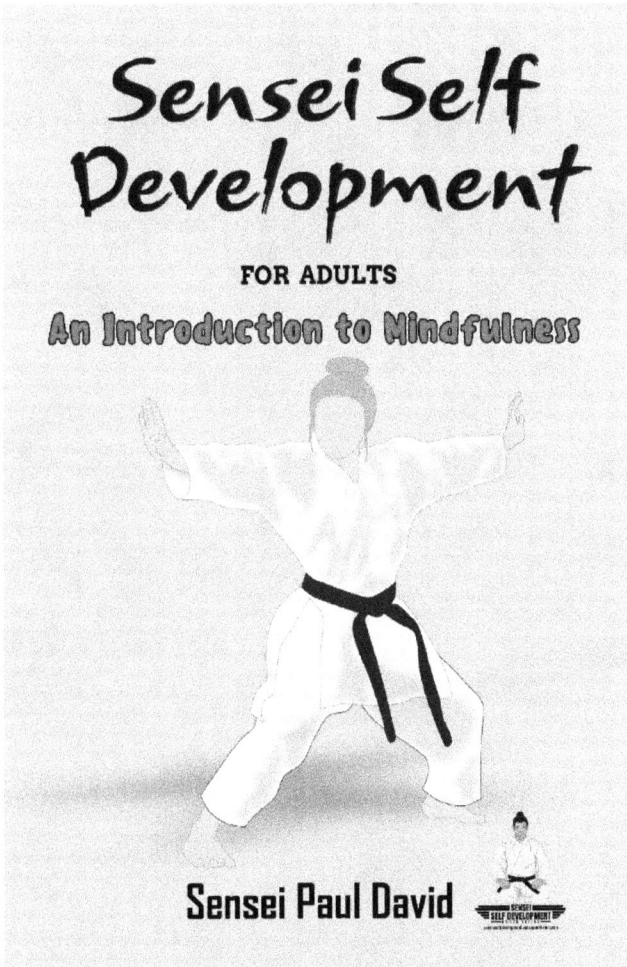

Check Out The SSD Chronicles Series CLICK HERE

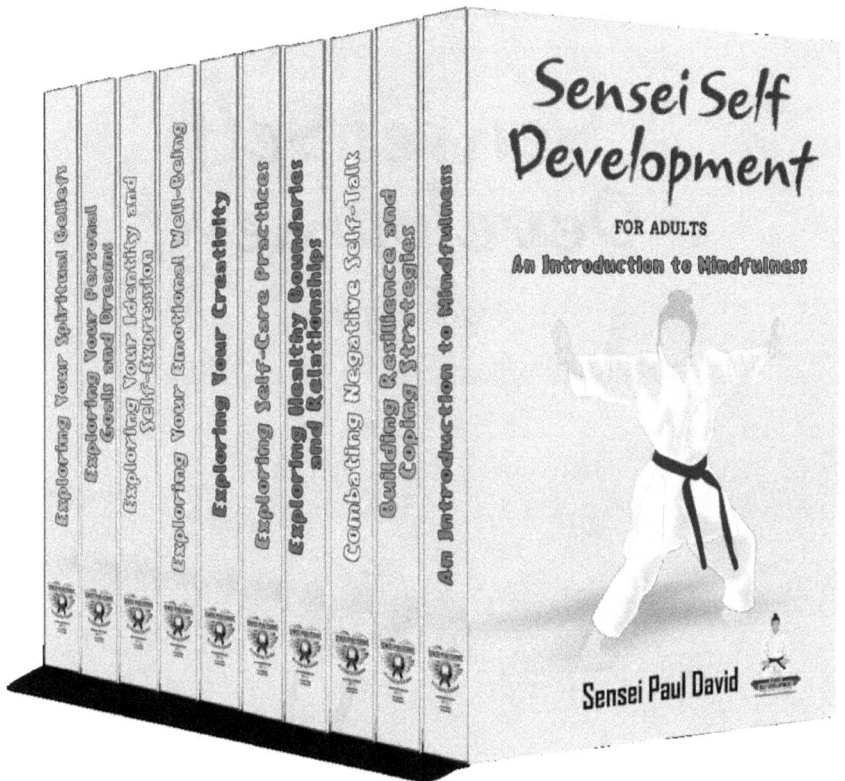

Exploring Your Spiritual Beliefs

Exploring Your Personal Goals and Dreams

Exploring Your Identity and Self-Expression

Exploring Your Emotional Well-Being

Exploring Your Creativity

Exploring Self-Care Practices

Exploring Healthy Boundaries and Relationships

Combatting Negative Self-Talk

Building Resilience and Coping Strategies

An Introduction to Mindfulness

Sensei Self Development

FOR ADULTS

An Introduction to Mindfulness

Sensei Paul David

Dedication

To those who courageously take action towards self-improvement - you are helping to evolve the world for generations to come.

- It's a great day to be alive!

If Found Please Contact:

_____

Reward If Found:

_____

MY COMMITMENT

I, _____

commit to writing This Sensei Self Development Journal for at least 10 days in a row, starting: _____

Writing this journal is valuable to me because:

_____

_____

_____

_____

_____

_____

If I finish a minimum of 10 consecutive days of writing in this journal, I will reward myself by:

_____

_____

_____

_____

_____

_____

If I don't finish 10 days of writing this journal, I will promise to:

_____

_____

_____

_____

_____

_____

I will do the following things to ensure that I write in my Sensei Self Development Journal every day:

_____

_____

_____

_____

_____

Get/Share Your FREE All-Ages Mental Health eBook Now at

www.senseiselfdevelopment.com

Or CLICK HERE

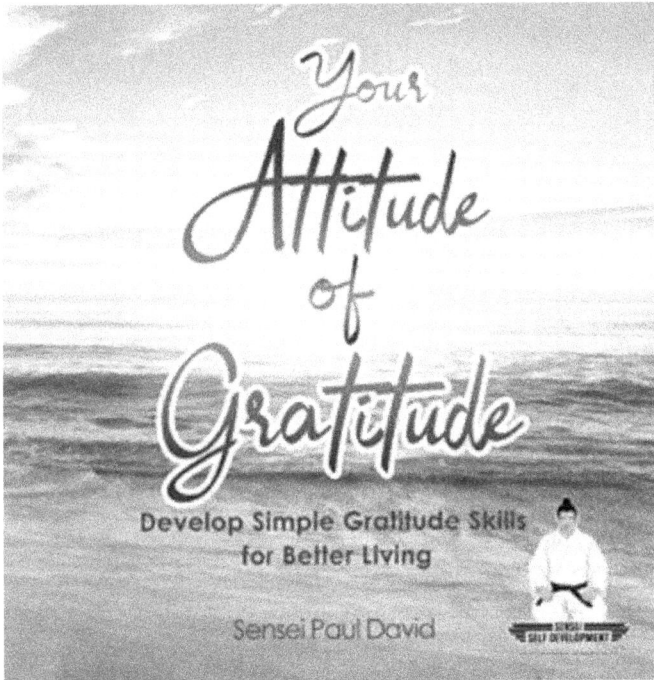

senseiselfdevelopment.com

Check Out Another Book In The
SSD BOOK SERIES:
senseipublishing.com/SSD_SERIES
CLICK HERE

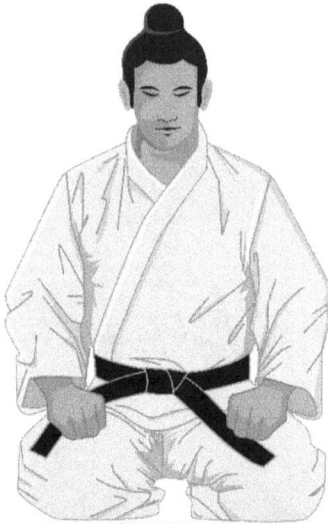

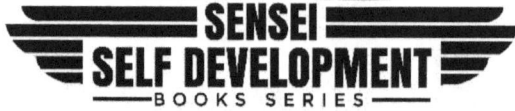

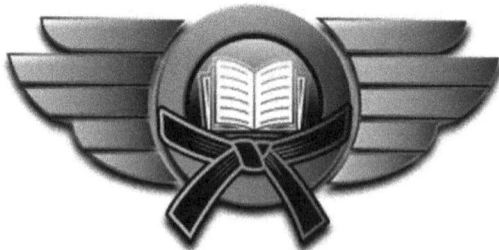

Join Our Publishing Journey!

If you would like to receive FUTURE FREE BOOKS and get to know us better, please click www.senseipublishing.com and join our newsletter by entering your email address in the pop-up box.

Follow Our Blog: senseipauldavid.ca

Follow/Like/Subscribe: Facebook, Instagram, YouTube:
@senseipublishing

Scan the QR Code with your phone or tablet

to follow us on social media: Like / Subscribe / Follow

A Message From The Author:
Sensei Paul David

Dear Reader,

Welcome to the world of mental health journaling – a sacred space for self-reflection, growth, and healing. Within these pages, you hold the power to uplift your spirit, invigorate your mind, and nourish your goals.

In a world that often moves at blink-and-you'll-miss-it speed, it's crucial to make time for self-care and self-discovery.

Anxiety, stress, and emotional turbulence may have clouded your mind, making it difficult to find clarity and peace within. But fear not! Together, we will navigate the labyrinth of emotions, and experiences, helping to simplify the path to mental well-being.

This journal is not merely a bunch of blank pages awaiting your words. It is your compassionate companion, offering solace and understanding during your unique journey. Here, you are free to unburden yourself, celebrate small and large victories, and confront the challenges that may still linger.

Within the sheltered realm of these pages, there is no judgment, no expectation, and no pressure. Your unique experience and perspective hold immeasurable worth, and your voice deserves to be heard. Whether you choose to fill the lines with eloquence or simply scribble fragments of your thoughts, please remember each entry is a valuable contribution to your growth.

In this sacred space, you are challenged to take off the mask we so often wear in the outside world. It is here that you can be raw, vulnerable, and authentic – allowing your true self to be seen and embraced without reservation. By giving yourself permission to explore the depths of your emotions and confront the shadows that may lurk within, you will discover profound insights and find the healing you seek over time.

As you embark on this journaling journey, I encourage you to embrace the process itself rather than fixate solely on the outcome. Remember, it is not about reaching a certain destination or ticking off boxes on a list of accomplishments. Rather, it is about cultivating self-awareness, fostering self-compassion, and nurturing a sense of curiosity about the intricate workings of your intelligently beautiful mind.

In the quiet moments of reflection, let your pen become a bridge between your inner world and the possibilities that lie ahead. Create a sanctuary for your thoughts, fears, triumphs, and dreams. As you pour your heart onto these pages, allow your words to be a living testament to courage, resilience, and an unwavering commitment to your own well-being.

I am honored to be a part of your journey, and I believe in your ability to navigate the twists and turns with grace and resilience. Remember, you are not alone in this – countless others have walked similar paths, faced similar challenges, and emerged stronger and wiser on the other side. You have the power to reclaim all of your untapped joy, cultivate a positive mindset that serves you, and foster a deep sense of self-love and peaceful confident. – And it will take a worth effort and time.

So, open the first page of this journal with hope, curiosity, and an open heart and open mind. Embrace the transformative power of self-reflection, and allow it to guide you towards a life of greater fulfilment and peace. Each journaling session is an opportunity to not only connect with yourself but also to rekindle the light within that sometimes flickers but never extinguishes.

Remember, the pages you are about to fill are not just a record of your journey but also a testament to your strength, resilience, and indomitable spirit. Cherish this space, invest in yourself, and let your words be an ode to the magnificent journey of becoming whole.

With great respect for your decision to evolve,

Paul

MY CONVICTION

Please circle your answers below

I am DECIDING to be patient with myself and this PROCESS each time I journal toward my improved state of mental well-being

YES   NO

"The present moment is filled with joy and happiness. If you are attentive, you will see it."

Thich Nhat Hanh

Introduction

Grief is a complex and completely normal reaction we experience when we face loss in our lives. It's a universal emotion, yet it's experienced uniquely by each person. Understanding grief helps in recognizing that the wide range of emotions you're feeling is normal and valid.

When we talk about grief, it's not just about feeling sad. It's about experiencing a whole spectrum of emotions that can sometimes feel conflicting or overwhelming. For instance, consider the loss of a loved one after a long-term illness. On one hand, there's a sense of relief that their suffering has ended, which is a positive and compassionate response. On the other hand, you're confronted with the profound sadness and emptiness of not being able to see or talk to them again. This duality of relief and pain is a classic example of how grief manifests.

But grief isn't limited to death. It can be triggered by a variety of life changes and losses. Divorce, for example, can bring a sense of freedom or release from a situation that was perhaps stressful or unhappy. At the same time, it might also bring about feelings of loneliness, fear of the unknown, or concerns about the future. This mix of liberation and anxiety is a natural part of the grieving process in the context of a relationship ending.

Beyond death and divorce, many situations can induce grief. These include:

- The death of a pet
- Moving to a new home or city
- Starting or finishing school,
- Major life events such as marriage or graduation.
- Overcoming addictions, which involves letting go of a substance or behavior that was once a significant part of one's life.
- Significant changes in health, which can alter one's lifestyle and sense of self.
- Retirement,

- The 'empty nest' phase, when children leave home.

Each of these situations involves a change in what was once familiar, comfortable, or significant.

Here, I will focus mainly on managing grief due to the loss of a loved one, but be aware that the process is the same for any kind of grief.

Grieving the Loss of a Loved One

When you lose someone close to you, it can feel like your entire world has shifted. The person you've lost was a significant part of your life, and their absence creates a profound void. In the wake of such a loss, it's common to long for their return, to hear their voice or see their smile just one more time. This yearning is a core part of grief.

During the grieving process, a wide array of emotions may surface. Sadness is often the most prominent, but it's not uncommon to feel alone or abandoned. Anger, too, can arise, sometimes directed at the circumstances, at others, or even at the person who has died for leaving you behind. These intense emotions can disrupt your daily life, affecting your ability to concentrate, complete tasks, or find restful sleep.

If you were caring for the person who passed away, the sudden end of this role could leave you feeling lost and directionless. The routines and responsibilities that once structured your day are gone, leaving you with unexpected and often uncomfortable stretches of unscheduled time.

Amidst these challenges, it's important to remember that there is no single correct way to mourn. Grief is a deeply personal experience, and each person navigates it in their own way. Some may find solace in solitude, while others may seek the company and support of friends and family.

Scientific studies on grief have expanded our understanding of how people cope with loss. Researchers have found that grief doesn't follow a linear path; instead, it can ebb and flow, sometimes unpredictably. This research emphasizes that there's no standard timeline or set of emotions that apply to everyone.

Cultural factors also significantly influence how people grieve. In some cultures, grief is expressed in quiet, private ways, while in others, it may involve public rituals and communal mourning. These cultural practices can also dictate the length of the mourning period and the types of behaviors that are considered appropriate during this time.

Experts in the field stress the importance of allowing yourself to experience your grief without judgment. People often fall into the trap of thinking they should feel or act a certain way during grief, but this can lead to additional emotional distress. Recognizing and accepting your emotions as they come is a crucial part of the healing process.

Grief is a natural part of the human experience, encompassing a range of emotions and reactions. It's important to keep in mind that grief:

- Is a normal response to loss
- can feel very much like fear

- Gradually it becomes more manageable.
- Requires time to process, often more than we or others might anticipate.
- Can feel intimidating or frightening at times.
- Might lead to dark thoughts, including depression or thoughts of suicide. While such thoughts can occur, it's important to discuss them with someone.
- Allows for moments of normalcy; it's okay to have times when you're not consumed by thoughts of the person who has passed.
- Doesn't mean you have to be hard on yourself. Be patient with your healing process and recognize when it's time to seek support.

The loss of someone close is a significant life event, and there's no quick way to adjust to such a change. Understanding and accepting the complexities of grief is crucial in navigating through this period.

Five Stages of Grief

When you're dealing with a big loss, like the death of someone close, you might go through different emotional stages. These stages were first described by Elisabeth Kübler-Ross and are really just a way to understand common feelings people have when they're grieving. It's normal to not go through all these stages or to experience them in a different order.

1. Denial: Right after a loss, it can be hard to accept what happened. This is denial. It's like your mind's way of not letting in too much pain all at once. You might think, "This can't be happening."

2. Anger: As the shock wears off, you might feel angry. This anger can be directed at anyone – the person who died, yourself, doctors, or even just the world. It's a way of dealing with the pain underneath.

3. Bargaining: Here, you might find yourself caught up in "What if" or "If only" thoughts. Like, "If only we had gone to the doctor sooner" or "What if I had been there." It's

a way of trying to regain control or make sense of the loss.

4. Depression: As reality sets in, you might feel very sad and even hopeless. You could have trouble sleeping, feel low on energy, or not want to do things you used to enjoy. It's different from clinical depression; it's more about feeling the full weight of the loss.

5. Acceptance: This doesn't mean you're okay with the loss, but rather that you understand it's a part of your life now. In this stage, emotions might stabilize, and you start figuring out how to live with this change.

Remember, these stages aren't rules. Everyone grieves differently. You might skip stages, experience them out of order, or revisit some stages multiple times. It's all about giving yourself space and time to feel what you need to feel.

How Long Does Grief Last

The duration and intensity of the grieving process can vary widely from one person to another, as each individual experiences grief in their own way.

Grief is often described in terms of stages, but for many, it feels more like a roller coaster ride with emotional highs and lows. This fluctuation can make it challenging for someone who is grieving to feel a sense of progress in coping with their loss. It's not unusual for a person to have periods of feeling better, only to find themselves feeling sad again later.

The question of how long the grieving process will last doesn't have a definitive answer. The duration and intensity of grief can be influenced by various factors, including the nature of the relationship with the deceased, the circumstances of their death, and the individual's personal life experiences.

It's common for the grieving process to extend over a year or more. This period is necessary for the individual to work through the emotional and life changes brought about by the loss of a loved one. While the intensity of the pain may lessen over time, it's normal to feel a connection to the deceased for many years.

Eventually, the grieving person can begin to redirect their emotional energy into other areas of life and strengthen other relationships.

The Ebb and Flow of Grief

Just as the ocean waves rise and fall, grief can bring alternating periods of intense emotions and calmer moments. In the early stages, like the high tide, the waves of grief can feel overwhelming, with deep and powerful emotions coming more frequently.

As time passes, these intense periods tend to become less consuming and shorter, similar to the way the tide gradually recedes. However, it's natural for the tide of grief to rise again during significant moments, like family weddings or the birth of a child, even years after the loss. These moments can bring back strong feelings, but they often don't last as long as they did in the beginning. The ebb and flow of grief is a process that evolves over time, reflecting the ongoing nature of our connection to what we have lost.

Symptoms of Grief

Grief manifests in various ways and can impact multiple aspects of life. Here are some common symptoms of grief:

1. Emotional Symptoms:

   - Sadness: A profound sense of sorrow is often the most immediate reaction.
   - Anger: Feelings of anger or frustration can arise, sometimes directed at the situation, oneself, or even the deceased.
   - Guilt: Guilt over things done or not done, or feeling guilty for surviving, is common.
   - Anxiety: Worry or anxiety about the future or the fear of facing life without a loved one.
   - Numbness: Emotional numbness or feeling detached from one's surroundings.

2. Physical Symptoms:

   - Fatigue: Feeling tired all the time or a lack of energy.
   - Sleep Disturbances: Difficulty falling or staying asleep, or sleeping too much.

- Changes in Appetite: Eating much more or less than usual.
- Physical Ailments: Headaches, stomachaches, or other physical symptoms with no apparent cause.

3. Cognitive Symptoms:

- Disbelief: Difficulty accepting the loss, feeling like it can't be real.
- Confusion: Trouble concentrating or making decisions.
- Preoccupation: Persistent thoughts about the loss or the person who has died.

4. Behavioral Symptoms:

- Withdrawal: Pulling away from social interactions or losing interest in activities previously enjoyed.
- Crying Spells: Frequent and intense periods of crying.
- Visiting Places or Carrying Objects: Going to places that remind one of the deceased or keeping their belongings close.

5. Social Symptoms:

- Feeling Isolated: Sensing that others cannot understand the depth of the loss.
- Changes in Relationships: Strained relationships or becoming closer to others who share the grief.

6. Spiritual Symptoms:

- Questioning Beliefs: Doubting one's spiritual beliefs or finding comfort in them.
- Searching for Meaning: Trying to make sense of the loss or finding a sense of purpose in it.

It's important to recognize that these symptoms are part of the natural grieving process. However, if they become overwhelming or persist for an extended period, seeking support from mental health professionals, support groups, or trusted individuals can be beneficial. Each person's experience with grief is unique, and the way symptoms manifest and are managed can vary widely.

How to Manage Grief

Trust the Process

Grief is a personal journey that can differ greatly from person to person. For some, it's a short and less intense experience, while for others, it can be a long and deeply painful process. Even when it seems like the grief has subsided, it's not uncommon for feelings of loss to resurface, especially during significant moments or reminders.

The key to navigating through grief is to trust and engage in the process, allowing yourself the time and space to experience these emotions. Suppressing or ignoring grief doesn't make it go away; instead, it's important to acknowledge and express your feelings. This could involve crying, talking about the loss, or participating in activities that help you remember the person.

You Won't Feel Like this Forever.

When you are in pain, it is easy to forget that that pain is temporary, and that it will ever stop. Keeping in mind that you won't feel this lethargic, this sad, and this fearful forever can make you resilient. It will instill hope in you. And hope is the antidote to chaos

You Will be Able to Handle it, Even if You Feel Like You Can't.

It's a natural instinct to want to steer clear of pain. When facing the loss of someone significant, the prospect of dealing with the grief can seem unbearable. However, it's with moving through these challenging experiences that we truly understand our ability to cope.

When we try to suppress or avoid our feelings of grief, they often return with greater intensity when triggered later on. Allowing ourselves to fully experience these difficult emotions is a way to build resilience. It helps in strengthening our inner resources and capabilities to handle life's challenges.

Seek Support

The intense pain of grief might make you feel like pulling away from people and withdrawing into yourself. However, getting support from others is crucial for healing after a loss. It's important to express your feelings during grief, even if you're usually someone who doesn't easily share emotions.

Sharing your experience of loss can lighten the weight of grief. This doesn't mean you always have to talk about your loss every time you're with friends and family. Sometimes, just being in the company of those who care about you can be comforting. The important thing is to avoid isolating yourself.

Now is the time to rely on friends and family. Even if you're used to being independent, it's okay to lean on others. Draw your friends and loved ones close, spend time with them, and accept their help. People often want to support you but may not know what you need, so it's helpful to communicate your needs, whether it's for a listening ear, a companion, or just a shoulder to cry on. If you feel you don't have someone to connect with, it's never too late to let people close to you.

Understand that many people might feel awkward or unsure about how to provide comfort during grief. Grieving can be a complex and daunting emotion for those who haven't experienced a similar loss. They may unintentionally say or do the wrong thing. However, it's important not to let this be a reason to retreat and avoid social interaction. If someone is reaching out to you, it's a sign of their care and concern.

Religion and spirituality

Religion and spirituality can offer profound comfort during the grieving process, serving as a source of solace for many. Engaging in specific religious rituals and rites can be a powerful way to bring people together, allowing them to share their grief and find support in community. Practices like sitting shiva, setting up a home altar, or annual gatherings at a cemetery are examples of how these traditions can help in the healing process. Attending religious services connects you to a community that's often ready to provide various forms of support, including a kind word, a listening ear, a shared meal, or acts of assistance, all of which can be incredibly comforting after a loss.

For some, religious or spiritual beliefs offer a larger perspective on life and death. The idea that a loved one is at peace, perhaps in heaven, or on another spiritual journey, can bring comfort. Beliefs such as being guided by the loved one in this life or being reunited after death can help maintain a sense of connection with the person who has passed.

If you find strength or solace in prayer, setting aside time for it can be beneficial. Reading spiritual texts, attending religious services, and discussing your feelings and the loss with a religious leader can also help place the experience within the context of your faith.

Apart from organized religion, finding solace in nature can also be therapeutic. Gardening or spending time in natural surroundings allows one to witness the cycles of life and death, offering a unique perspective and comfort. Likewise, practices like meditation and yoga can provide a sense of peace and help in managing grief. These activities offer quiet reflection and a chance to connect with one's inner thoughts and feelings.

Common Humanity

In grief, we're all the same. It hits everyone. It doesn't matter where you're from, what you do, or how strong you think you are. We all feel that ache, that missing piece. It's part of being human. We lose, we hurt, we heal. It's a cycle everyone knows. It's not just your story, it's everyone's at some point. That's the thing about grief – it's a shared experience, even if it feels lonely. It reminds us that we're all in this together, going through the same motions of being human.

Remembering this shared aspect of grief can be a source of comfort. Knowing you're not alone in your pain, that others have felt this too and found their way through, can make the burden a little lighter. It's a reminder that just as others have healed, you too have the strength to cope and heal in time. This sense of shared humanity brings a glimmer of hope in the darkest times, reminding us that grief, while personal, is also a path walked by many.

Honor Your Loved One

Honoring a loved one through creativity or meaningful activities can be a powerful part of the healing process after a loss. This act of remembrance and expression can take many forms, depending on what feels right for you.

Creating artwork is one way to channel your feelings and memories into something tangible. This could be a painting or drawing that captures a special moment, a sculpture that represents something your loved one cherished, or even a collage of photos and mementos. The act of creating something not only serves as a tribute to the person you've lost but also offers a therapeutic outlet for your emotions.

Gathering with friends and family to share memories is another beautiful way to honor your loved one. This could be a formal gathering or a casual get-together where everyone shares stories, anecdotes, and the positive impact the deceased had on their lives. Such gatherings not only celebrate the life of the person you're mourning but also strengthen the bonds among those who share in your grief.

These acts of creative expression and shared remembrance help keep the memory of your loved one alive in a meaningful way. They allow you to process your grief while also celebrating the unique life and legacy of the person you miss. Each story told, each piece created, becomes a part of the tapestry of memories that you carry with you, a testament to the love and connection that continue beyond loss.

Journaling

Writing or journaling can be a highly effective way to navigate through grief, especially when you find it hard to verbalize your feelings. It's a personal space where you can pour out your thoughts, emotions, and memories without fear of judgment or expectation. When overwhelmed or uncertain about what to write, guided prompts can be incredibly helpful.

Guided grief journaling involves using specific prompts that lead you through the process of exploring and expressing your emotions. These prompts can vary from simple questions like

"What are you feeling today?" to more in-depth ones like "Write about a favorite memory with your loved one." They offer a structured way to reflect on your feelings and experiences, making the blank page less daunting.

Research supports the effectiveness of this method. One study indicated that people who engaged in guided grief journaling experienced long-term improvements in dealing with their grief. This kind of journaling helps not just in expressing immediate emotions but also in processing the loss over time. It can lead to greater self-awareness, a clearer understanding of your personal grief journey, and eventually, a path towards healing.

Whether it's just a few lines a day or pages of memories and reflections, journaling offers a safe and private outlet for your grief.

Talk to a Counselor

If you find that your grief is overwhelming and difficult to manage, it might be beneficial to talk to a therapist or grief counselor. Seeking a mental health professional who specializes in grief counseling can provide you with the support and guidance needed to navigate through intense emotions. An experienced therapist can help you address and work through the challenges you're facing in your grieving process, offering strategies and insights to cope with the pain and move forward.

Take Care of Yourself

Taking care of yourself is incredibly important while you're grieving. It's essential to pay attention to basic health and self-care practices during this time.

1. Eating Well: A balanced diet is crucial. It can help you cope better with the stress of grief. Try to include a variety of vegetables, fruits, and lean proteins in your meals. Drinking plenty of water is also important. If you find you're not very hungry, eat smaller meals more often throughout the day.

2. Taking Medications: Grief can weaken your immune system and make you more susceptible to illness. If you have

prescribed medications, it's important to continue taking them as directed.

3. Sleeping Well: Grief often leads to exhaustion, so maintaining a regular sleep schedule is key. If you're feeling tired during the day, a short nap of about 20 minutes can be refreshing. Be cautious with caffeine and alcohol, as they can disrupt your sleep at night. If you're struggling with ongoing insomnia, it might be a good idea to talk to your doctor.

4. Regular Exercise: Keeping up with, or starting, an exercise routine can be very beneficial. Whether it's sticking to your usual exercise regimen or engaging in gentle activities like walking, cycling, or yoga, physical activity can provide a distraction.

Focusing on these aspects of self-care can help you navigate the grieving process more effectively, providing your body and mind with the support they need during this challenging time.

Take Care of Others

Taking care of others who are grieving can provide a sense of purpose and fulfillment, and it also offers much-needed support to the person who is mourning. When you step in to help someone dealing with loss, it can strengthen your connection with them and also bring a sense of satisfaction in knowing you're making a difference during a difficult time.

Listening is one of the most valuable things you can do. Just being there, offering a shoulder to cry on, or an ear to listen to their memories and feelings can mean a lot. This emotional support allows them to feel understood and not alone in their grief.

Helping with everyday tasks can also be a great way to show care. This might mean running errands, helping with household chores, or preparing meals. These acts of service can lighten their load, allowing them more space to grieve and heal.

Encouraging self-care is another way to support them. It can be as simple as inviting them for a walk, joining in a hobby, or cooking a healthy meal together. This not only helps them look after their well-being but also provides opportunities for you to spend quality time together.

Sometimes, offering a distraction or a break from the intensity of grief can be helpful. This could involve planning a small outing, watching a movie together, or engaging in a light-hearted activity. These moments can provide a brief respite from grief for both of you.

Taking care of someone who is grieving is not just about helping them; it's also about creating a meaningful experience for yourself. It reinforces the value of connection, empathy, and kindness, and these actions can be deeply rewarding for both parties involved.

Before We Get Started…

Remember, mindfulness journaling is a personal practice, and these questions are meant to guide and inspire you. Feel free to adapt and modify them to suit your needs and preferences. Explore, reflect, and embrace the opportunity to deepen your self-awareness and cultivate a sense of inner peace.

Date ___ / ___ / ___ : S M T W Th F S

I feel:
(please circle)

because   because   because   because   because
_____ _____ _____ _____ _____
_____ _____ _____ _____ _____

Today I Am Grateful For

1. _____
2. _____
3. _____

What could help transform today into a remarkable day?

Reflective Writing

What spiritual beliefs do you currently hold?

_____

_____

_____

_____

_____

_____

_____

_____

_____

What is grief?

a) The feeling of sadness or loss after a physical injury

b) The emotional response to losing a loved one or something significant

c) A mental disorder characterized by extreme sadness and hopelessness

d) The aftermath of a natural disaster or traumatic event

All Are Correct - Choose The Response You Feel Is Most Important To Remember

Date ___/___/___: S   M   T   W   Th   F   S

I feel:
(please circle)

because   because   because   because   because
_____   _____   _____   _____   _____
_____   _____   _____   _____   _____

Today I Am Grateful For

1. _____
2. _____
3. _____

What could help transform today into a remarkable day?

Reflective Writing

How has your spiritual beliefs evolved since you were a child?

_____

_____

_____

_____

_____

_____

_____

Which of the following is NOT a stage of grief according to the Kübler-Ross model?

a) Denial
b) Bargaining
c) Acceptance
d) Compromise

All Are Correct - Choose The Response You Feel Is Most Important To Remember

Date ___ / ___ / ___ : S M T W Th F S

I feel:
(please circle)

because _____ because _____ because _____ because _____ because _____

Today I Am Grateful For

1. _____
2. _____
3. _____

What could help transform today into a remarkable day?

Reflective Writing

Do you feel that your spiritual beliefs have a strong influence on your life?

_____

_____

_____

_____

_____

_____

_____

_____

How long does the grief process usually last?

a) A few weeks to a month
b) 6-12 months
c) 2-5 years
d) The grief process varies for each individual and can last a lifetime.

All Are Correct - Choose The Response You Feel Is Most Important To Remember

Date ___ / ___ / ___ : S   M   T   W   Th   F   S

I feel:
(please circle)

because   because   because   because   because
_____   _____   _____   _____   _____
_____   _____   _____   _____   _____

Today I Am Grateful For

1. _____
2. _____
3. _____

What could help transform today into a remarkable day?

Reflective Writing

What spiritual experiences have you had that have changed your beliefs?

_____

_____

_____

_____

_____

_____

_____

What is the difference between grief and mourning?

a) Grief is the emotional response, while mourning is the outward expression of grief.
b) Grief is experienced after the death of a loved one, while mourning is experienced after the loss of a job.
c) Grief is a natural human emotion, while mourning is a learned behavior.
d) Grief is a personal experience, while mourning is a cultural or societal response.

All Are Correct - Choose The Response You Feel Is Most Important To Remember

Date ___ / ___ / ___ : S   M   T   W   Th   F   S

I feel:
(please circle)

because   because   because   because   because
_____   _____   _____   _____   _____
_____   _____   _____   _____   _____

Today I Am Grateful For

1. _____
2. _____
3. _____

What could help transform today into a remarkable day?

Reflective Writing

Do you feel that the spiritual path you are on is meaningful or fulfilling to you?

_____

_____

_____

_____

_____

_____

_____

Which of the following could be a physical symptom of grief?

a) Increased appetite
b) Insomnia
c) Decreased heart rate
d) Increased energy levels

All Are Correct - Choose The Response You Feel Is Most Important To Remember

Date ___ / ___ / ___ : S M T W Th F S

I feel:
(please circle)

:) because _____
:D because _____
:) because _____
:(because _____
>:(because _____

Today I Am Grateful For

1. _____
2. _____
3. _____

What could help transform today into a remarkable day?

Reflective Writing

What sources do you rely on for guidance or understanding when exploring your spiritual beliefs?

_____

_____

_____

_____

_____

_____

_____

What is complex grief?

a) Grief that lasts longer than a year
b) Grief that occurs after the loss of a pet
c) Grief that is accompanied by intense guilt or anger
d) Grief that is experienced by children only

All Are Correct - Choose The Response You Feel Is Most Important To Remember

Date ___ / ___ / ___ : S   M   T   W   Th   F   S

I feel:
(please circle)

because   because   because   because   because
_____ _____ _____ _____ _____
_____ _____ _____ _____ _____

Today I Am Grateful For

1. _____
2. _____
3. _____

What could help transform today into a remarkable day?

Reflective Writing

How do you feel when you practice your spiritual beliefs?

_____

_____

_____

_____

_____

_____

_____

What are some examples of unhealthy coping mechanisms for grief?

a) Seeking support from friends and family
b) Engaging in unhealthy behaviors, such as excessive drinking or drug use
c) Joining a support group
d) Writing in a grief journal

All Are Correct - Choose The Response You Feel Is Most Important To Remember

41

Date ___ / ___ / ___ : S M T W Th F S

I feel:
(please circle)

because _____ because _____ because _____ because _____ because _____

Today I Am Grateful For
1. _____
2. _____
3. _____

What could help transform today into a remarkable day?

Reflective Writing

How do you differentiate between spiritual beliefs and religious beliefs?

_____

_____

_____

_____

_____

_____

_____

What is anticipatory grief?

a) Grief that is experienced after the loss of a loved one
b) Grief that is experienced before a loved one passes away
c) Grief that is experienced during the acceptance stage
d) Grief that is experienced in childhood

All Are Correct - Choose The Response You Feel Is Most Important To Remember

Date ___ / ___ / ___ : S M T W Th F S

I feel:
(please circle)

because   because   because   because   because
_____   _____   _____   _____   _____
_____   _____   _____   _____   _____

Today I Am Grateful For

1. _____
2. _____
3. _____

What could help transform today into a remarkable day?

Reflective Writing

How important is it to you to find alignment
between your spiritual beliefs and your actions?

_____

_____

_____

_____

_____

_____

_____

Which of the following could be a sign of unresolved grief?

a) Talking frequently about the loss
b) Engaging in self-care activities
c) Avoiding reminders or triggers of the loss
d) Seeking counseling or therapy

All Are Correct - Choose The Response You Feel Is Most Important To Remember

Date ___/___/___: S M T W Th F S

I feel: because   because   because   because   because
(please circle)   _____ _____ _____ _____ _____

Today I Am Grateful For

1. _____
2. _____
3. _____

What could help transform today into a remarkable day?

Reflective Writing

What is the role of meditation in your spiritual journey?

_____

_____

_____

_____

_____

_____

_____

How can friends and family members best support someone who is grieving?

a) By avoiding the topic of the loss
b) By offering platitudes like "time heals all wounds"
c) By listening and being present for the person
d) By ignoring any negative emotions the person may be feeling

All Are Correct - Choose The Response You Feel Is Most Important To Remember

Date ___ / ___ / ___: S   M   T   W   Th   F   S

I feel:
(please circle)

because   because   because   because   because

_____ _____ _____ _____ _____

_____ _____ _____ _____ _____

Today I Am Grateful For

1. _____
2. _____
3. _____

What could help transform today into a remarkable day?

Reflective Writing

What spiritual practices do you incorporate into your daily life?

_____

_____

_____

_____

_____

_____

_____

How can children effectively cope with grief?

a) By suppressing their emotions
b) By talking to a therapist or counselor
c) By engaging in unhealthy behaviors
d) By ignoring the loss and focusing on other things

All Are Correct - Choose The Response You Feel Is Most Important To Remember

Date ___ / ___ / ___ : S   M   T   W   Th   F   S

I feel:
(please circle)

because   because   because   because   because
_____ _____ _____ _____ _____
_____ _____ _____ _____ _____

Today I Am Grateful For

1. _____
2. _____
3. _____

What could help transform today into a remarkable day?

Reflective Writing

Do you have any rituals or traditions that you
follow as part of your spiritual practice?

_____

_____

_____

_____

_____

_____

_____

_____

What is disenfranchised grief?

a) Grief that is experienced by the disenfranchised population
b) Grief that is experienced by the LGBTQ+ community
c) Grief that is not openly acknowledged or supported by society
d) Grief that is experienced after a miscarriage or stillbirth

All Are Correct - Choose The Response You Feel Is Most Important To Remember

Date ___ / ___ / ___ : S M T W Th F S

I feel:
(please circle)

because _____ because _____ because _____ because _____ because _____

Today I Am Grateful For
1. _____
2. _____
3. _____

What could help transform today into a remarkable day?

Reflective Writing
What is the most meaningful spiritual experience you have ever had?

_____

_____

_____

_____

_____

_____

_____

_____

How can employers support grieving employees?

a) By expecting them to return to work immediately after a loss
b) By offering a flexible work schedule
c) By not acknowledging the employee's loss
d) By providing adequate bereavement leave

All Are Correct - Choose The Response You Feel Is Most Important To Remember

Date ___ / ___ / ___: S   M   T   W   Th   F   S

I feel: (please circle)

because   because   because   because   because

_____ _____ _____ _____ _____

_____ _____ _____ _____ _____

Today I Am Grateful For

1. _____

2. _____

3. _____

What could help transform today into a remarkable day?

Reflective Writing

How do you balance your spiritual practice with the demands of everyday life?

_____

_____

_____

_____

_____

_____

_____

What is the role of spirituality in grief?

a) It has no impact on the grieving process
b) It can provide comfort and a sense of purpose for some individuals
c) It can worsen feelings of grief and guilt
d) It only applies to individuals who are religious

All Are Correct - Choose The Response You Feel Is Most Important To Remember

Date ___ / ___ / ___: S   M   T   W   Th   F   S

I feel:
(please circle)

because   because   because   because   because
_____   _____   _____   _____   _____
_____   _____   _____   _____   _____

Today I Am Grateful For

1. _____
2. _____
3. _____

What could help transform today into a remarkable day?

Reflective Writing

What advice would you give to someone just beginning to explore their spiritual beliefs?

_____

_____

_____

_____

_____

_____

_____

What is the purpose of a grief support group?

a) To provide a safe space for individuals to share their grief with others who understand
b) To pressure individuals into expressing their emotions
c) To skip over the grieving process and find closure immediately
d) To force individuals to confront their loss before they are ready

All Are Correct - Choose The Response You Feel Is Most Important To Remember

As we reach the final pages of this journey through "Positive Mindset," I want to extend my heartfelt thanks to you. Your commitment to exploring positivity and its transformative power is not only commendable but a testament to your desire for personal growth and a richer, more fulfilling life experience.

Remember, the journey towards a positive mindset is ongoing and ever-evolving. Each day presents new opportunities to apply these principles, to learn, and to grow. I encourage you to revisit these pages whenever you need a reminder of your incredible potential to foster positivity and resilience in the face of life's challenges.

As we part ways, I leave you with a quote that has been a guiding star in my journey: "The greatest discovery of any generation is that a human can alter his life by altering his attitude."

— William James.

Thank you for allowing me to be a part of your journey. May your path be filled with light, hope, and endless possibilities. Farewell, and may you carry the spirit of positivity with you, today and always.

With gratitude and best wishes,

Sensei Paul David

Reflective Writing

The End

As you close the pages of this mindfulness journal, remember that each word you've written is a step on your journey towards self-awareness and inner peace. Embrace the moments of clarity, the revelations, and even the uncertainties you've encountered along the way. Let this journal be a testament to your growth and a reminder that every day offers a new opportunity to be present, to observe, and to appreciate the simple wonders of life. Carry these lessons forward, and may your path be filled with mindful moments and serene reflections. Until we meet again in these pages, be gentle with yourself and stay anchored in the now.

Mindfulness isn't difficult, we just need to remember to do it.

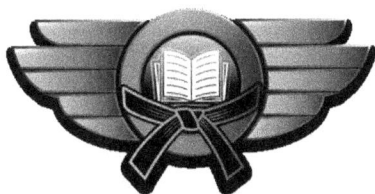

Thank You!

If you found this book helpful, I would be grateful if you would **post an honest review on Amazon** so this book can reach other supportive readers like you!

All you need to do is digitally flip to the back and leave your review. Or visit amazon.com/author/senseipauldavid click the correct book cover and click on the blue link next to the yellow stars that say, "customer reviews."

As always...
It's a great day to be alive!

Get/Share Your FREE SSD Mental Health Chronicles at
www.senseiselfdevelopment.care

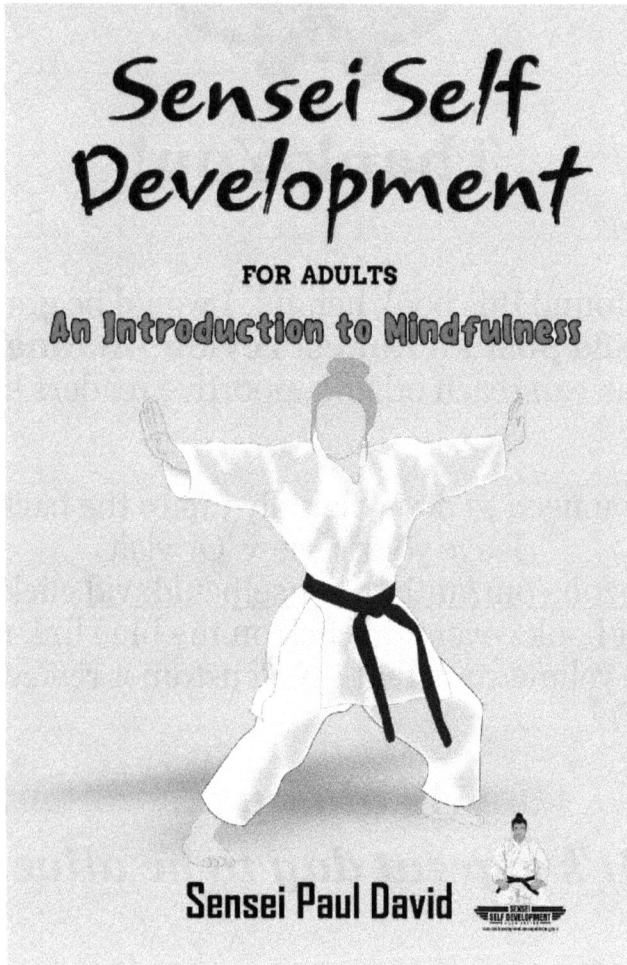

Sensei Self Development

FOR ADULTS

An Introduction to Mindfulness

Sensei Paul David

Check Out The SSD Chronicles
Series CLICK HERE

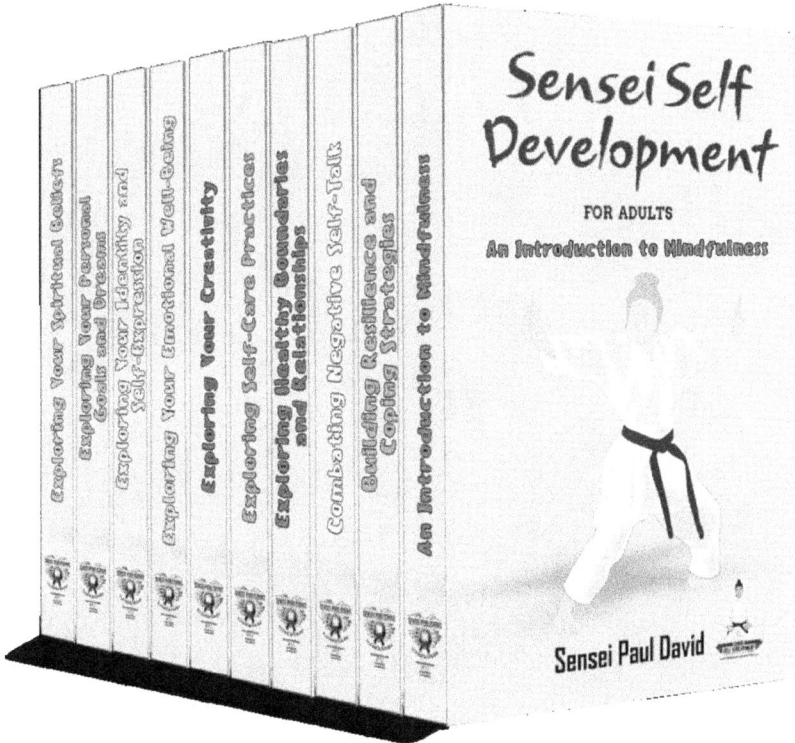

Exploring Your Spiritual Beliefs

Exploring Your Personal Goals and Dreams

Exploring Your Identity and Self-Expression

Exploring Your Emotional Well-Being

Exploring Your Creativity

Exploring Self-Care Practices

Exploring Healthy Boundaries and Relationships

Combatting Negative Self-Talk

Building Resilience and Coping Strategies

An Introduction to Mindfulness

Sensei Self Development

FOR ADULTS

An Introduction to Mindfulness

Sensei Paul David

Get/Share Your FREE All-Ages Mental Health eBook Now at

www.senseiselfdevelopment.com

Or CLICK HERE

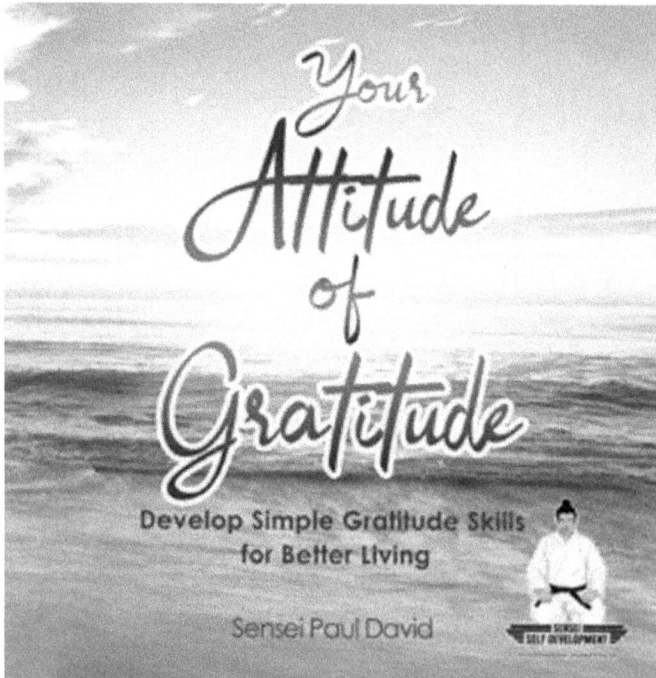

senseiselfdevelopment.com

Click Another Book In The SSD BOOK SERIES:

senseipublishing.com/SSD_SERIES

CLICK HERE

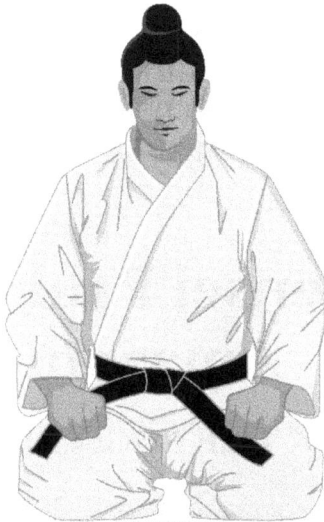

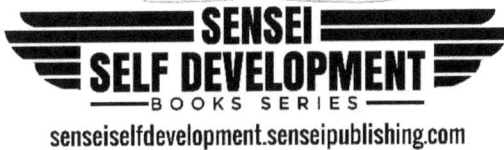

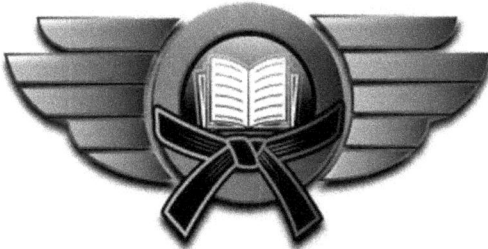

Join Our Publishing Journey!

If you would like to receive FREE BOOKS, please visit **www.senseipublishing.com**. Join our newsletter by entering your email address in the pop-up box

Follow Sensei Paul David on Amazon

CLICK THE LOGO BELOW

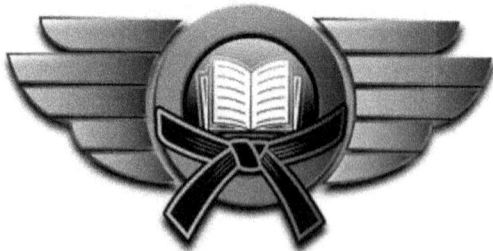

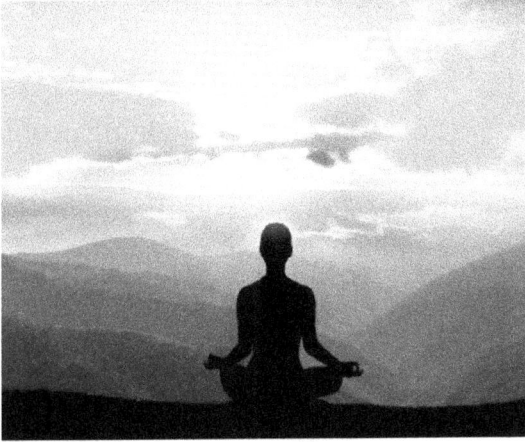

FREE BONUS!!!
Experience Over 25 FREE Engaging Guided Meditations!

Prized Skills & Practices for Adults & Kids. Help Restore Deep-Sleep, Lower Stress, Improve Posture, Navigate Uncertainty & More.

Download the Free Insight Timer App and click the link below:
http://insig.ht/sensei_paul

About Sensei Publishing

Sensei Publishing commits itself to helping people of all ages transform into better versions of themselves by providing high-quality and research-based self-development books with an emphasis on mental health and guided meditations. Sensei Publishing offers well-written e-books, audiobooks, paperbacks and online courses that simplify complicated but practical topics in line with its mission to inspire people towards positive transformation.

It's a great day to be alive!

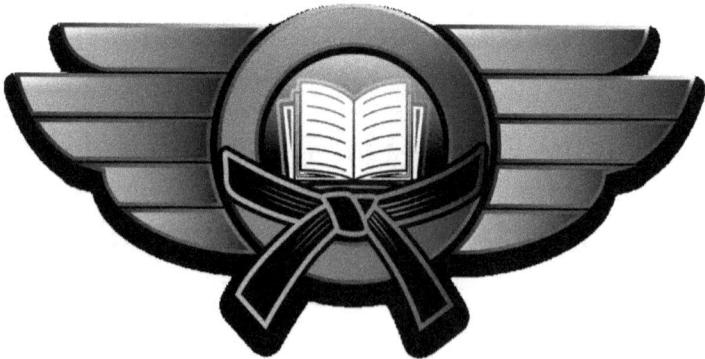

About the Author

I create simple & transformative eBooks & Guided Meditations for Adults & Children proven to help navigate uncertainty, solve niche problems & bring families closer together.

I'm a former finance project manager, private pilot, jiu-jitsu instructor, musician & former University of Toronto Fitness Trainer. I prefer a science-based approach to focus on these & other areas in my life to stay humble & hungry to evolve. I hope you enjoy my work and I'd love to hear your feedback.

- It's a great day to be alive!

Sensei Paul David

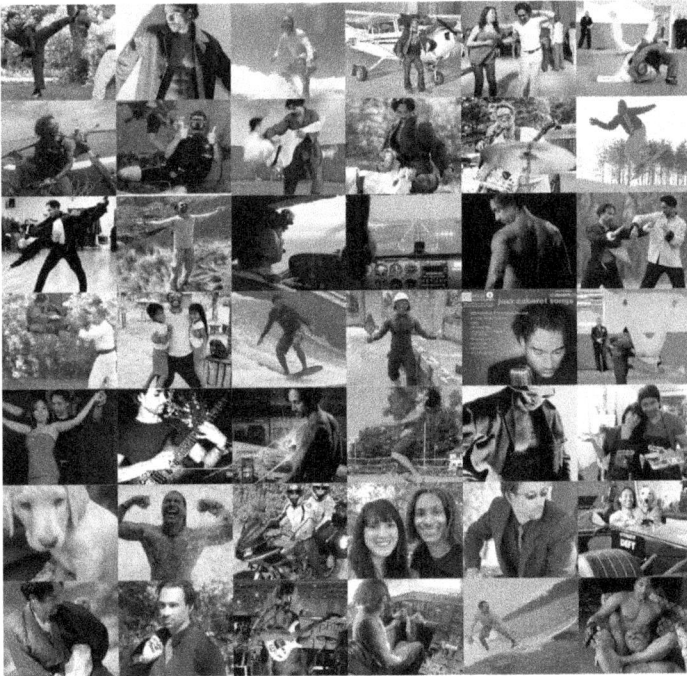

Scan & Follow/Like/Subscribe: Facebook, Instagram,
YouTube: @senseipublishing

Scan using your phone/iPad camera for Social Media
Visit us at www.senseipublishing.com and sign up for our
newsletter to learn more about our exciting books and to
experience our FREE Guided Meditations for Kids & Adults.

www.ingramcontent.com/pod-product-compliance
Lightning Source LLC
Chambersburg PA
CBHW071244020426
42333CB00015B/1626